# The Ultimate Intermittent Fasting Cookbook

*Quick, Easy and Inexpensive Recipes to Lose Weight Fast (for Both Men and Women)*

**Dotty Rivers**

**Diet Acclaimed Press**

# CONTENTS

iii

# BREAKFAST

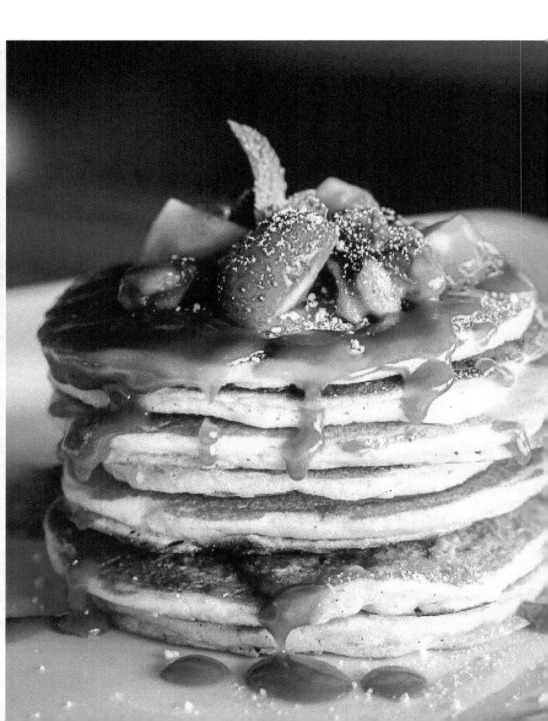

# Pizza Hack

**Prep Time:** 5-10 minutes

**Cook Time:** 15-20 minutes

**Serves:** 1

**What you need:**

- 1/4 fueling of garlic mashed potato
- 1/2 egg whites
- 1/4 tablespoon of baking powder
- 3/4 oz. of reduced-fat shredded mozzarella
- 1/8 cup of sliced white mushrooms
- /16 cup of pizza sauce
- 3/4 oz. of ground beef
- 1/4 sliced black olives
- You also need a sauté pan, baking sheets, and parchment paper

**Steps:**

1. Start by preheating the oven to 400°.
2. Mix your baking powder and garlic potato packet.
3. Add egg whites to your mixture and stir well until it blends.
4. Line the baking sheet with parchment paper and pour the mixed batter onto it.
5. Put another parchment paper on top of the batter and spread out the batter to a 1/8-inch circle.
6. Then place another baking sheet on top; this way, the batter is between two baking sheets.
7. Place into an oven and bake for about 8 minutes until the pizza crust is golden brown.

8. For the toppings, place your ground beef in a sauté pan and fry till it's brown and wash your mushrooms very well.

9. After the crust is baked, remove the top layer of parchment paper carefully to prevent the foam from sticking to the pizza crust.

10. Put your toppings on top of the crust and bake for an extra 8 minutes.

11. Once ready, slide the pizza off the parchment paper and onto a plate.

**Nutrition**:

Calories: 478

Protein: 30 g

Carbohydrates: 22 g

Fats: 29 g

# Amaranth Porridge

**Prep Time:** 5 minutes

**Cook Time:** 30 minutes

**Serves:** 2.

- What you need:
- 2 cups coconut milk
- 2 cups alkaline water
- 1 cup amaranth
- 2 tbsps. coconut oil
- 1 tbsp. ground cinnamon

**Steps:**

1. In a saucepan, mix in the milk with water, then boil the mixture.
2. You stir in the amaranth, then reduce the heat to medium.
3. Cook on the medium heat, then simmer for at least 30 minutes as you stir it occasionally.
4. Turn off the heat.
5. Add in cinnamon and coconut oil then stir.
6. Serve.

**Nutrition:**

Calories: 434 kcal

Fat: 35g

Carbs: 27g

Protein: 6.7g

# Pancakes with Berries

**Prep Time:** 5 minutes

**Cook Time:** 20 minutes

**Serves:** 2

**What you need:**

- Pancake:

- 1 egg

- 50 g ~~spelled~~ spelt flour

- 50 g almond flour

- 15 g coconut flour

- 150 ml of water

- salt

Filling:

- 40 g mixed berries

- 10 g chocolate

- 5 g powdered sugar

- 4 tbsp yogurt

**Steps:**

1. Put the flour, egg, and some salt in a blender jar.

2. Add 150 ml of water.

3. Mix everything with a whisk.

4. Mix everything into a batter.

5. Heat a coated pan.

6. Put in half of the batter.

7. Once the pancake is firm, turn it over.

8. Take out the pancake, add the second half of the batter to the pan and repeat.

9. Melt chocolate over a water bath.

10. Let the pancakes cool.

11. Brush the pancakes with the yogurt.

12. Wash the berry and let it drain.

13. Put berries on the yogurt.

14. Roll up the pancakes.

15. Sprinkle them with the powdered sugar.

16. Decorate the whole thing with the melted chocolate.

**Nutrition:**

kcal: 298

Carbohydrates: 26 g

Protein: 21 g

Fat: 9 g

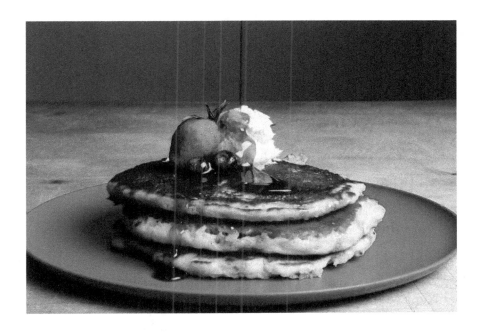

# Omelette à la Margherita

**Prep Time:** 10 minutes

**Cook Time:** 20 minutes

**Serves:** 2

**What you need:**

- 3 eggs
- 50 g parmesan cheese
- 2 tbsp heavy cream
- 1 tbsp olive oil
- 1 teaspoon oregano
- nutmeg
- salt
- pepper
- For covering:
- 3 - 4 stalks of basil
- 1 tomato
- 100 g grated mozzarella

**Steps:**

1. Mix the cream and eggs in a medium bowl.
2. Add the grated parmesan, nutmeg, oregano, pepper and salt and stir everything.
3. Heat the oil in a pan.
4. Add 1/2 of the egg and cream to the pan.
5. Let the omelette set over medium heat, turn it, and then remove it.
6. Repeat with the second half of the egg mixture.

7. Cut the tomatoes into slices and place them on top of the omelets.

8. Scatter the mozzarella over the tomatoes.

9. Place the omelets on a baking sheet.

10. Cook at 180 degrees for 5 to 10 minutes.

11. Then take the omelets out and decorate them with the basil leaves.

**Nutrition:**

kcal: 402

Carbohydrates: 7 g

Protein: 21 g

Fat: 34 g

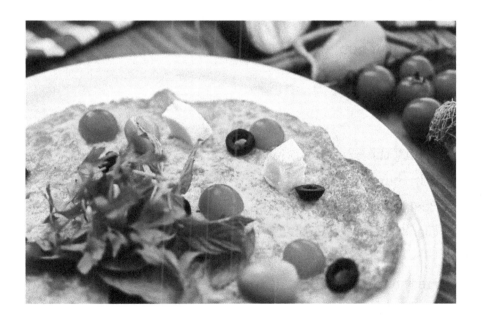

# Omelette With Tomatoes and Spring Onions

**Prep Time:** 5 minutes

**Cook Time:** 20 minutes

**Serves:**

**What you need:**

- 6 eggs
- 2 tomatoes
- 2 spring onions
- 1 shallot
- 2 tbsp butter
- 1 tbsp olive oil
- 1 pinch of nutmeg
- salt
- pepper

**Steps:**

1. Whisk the eggs in a bowl.
2. Mix them and season them with salt and pepper.
3. Peel the shallot and chop it up.
4. Clean the onions and cut them into rings.
5. Wash the tomatoes and cut them into pieces.
6. Heat butter and oil in a pan.
7. Braise half of the shallots in it.
8. Add half the egg mixture.
9. Let everything set over medium heat.
10. Scatter a few tomatoes and onion rings on top.

11. Repeat with the second half of the egg mixture.

12. At the end, spread the grated nutmeg over the whole thing.

**Nutrition:**

kcal: 263

Carbohydrates: 8 g

Protein: 20.3 g

Fat: 24 g

# Coconut Chia Pudding with Berries

**Prep Time:** 20 minutes

**Cook Time:** 45 minutes

**Serves:** 2

**What you need:**

- 150 g raspberries and blueberries
- 60 g chia seeds
- 500 ml coconut milk
- 1 teaspoon agave syrup
- ½ teaspoon ground bourbon vanilla

**Steps:**

1. Put the chia seeds, agave syrup, and vanilla in a bowl.
2. Pour in the coconut milk.
3. Mix thoroughly and let it soak for 30 minutes.
4. Meanwhile, wash the berries and let them drain well.
5. Divide the coconut chia pudding between two glasses.
6. Put the berries on top.

**Nutrition:**

kcal: 662

Carbohydrates: 18 g

Protein: 8 g

Fat: 55 g

# Eel on Scrambled Eggs and Bread

**Prep Time:** 5 minutes

**Cook Time:** 10 minutes

**Serves:** 2

**What you need:**

- 4 eggs
- 1 shallot
- 4 slices of low carb bread
- 2 sticks of dill
- 200 g smoked eel
- 1 tbsp oil
- salt
- White pepper

**Steps:**

1. Mix the eggs in a bowl and season with salt and pepper.
2. Peel the shallot and cut it into fine cubes.
3. Chop the dill.
4. Remove the skin from the eel and cut it into pieces.
5. Heat the oil in a pan and steam the shallot in it.
6. Add in the eggs in and let them set.
7. Use the spatula to turn the eggs several times.
8. Reduce the heat and add the dill.

9. Stir everything.

10. Spread the scrambled eggs over four slices of bread.

11. Put the eel pieces on top.

12. Add some fresh dill and serve everything.

**Nutrition:**

kcal: 830

Carbohydrates: 8 g

Protein: 45 g

Fat: 64 g

# Chia Seed Gel with Pomegranate and Nuts

**Prep Time:** 5 minutes

**Cook Time:** 10 minutes

**Serves:** 3

**What you need:**

- 20 g hazelnuts
- 20 g walnuts
- 120 ml almond milk
- 4 tbsp chia seeds
- 4 tbsp pomegranate seeds
- 1 teaspoon agave syrup
- Some lime juices

**Steps:**

1. Finely chop the nuts.

2. Mix the almond milk with the chia seeds.

3. Let everything soak for 10 to 20 minutes.

4. Occasionally stir the mixture with the chia seeds.

5. Stir in the agave syrup.

6. Pour 2 tablespoons of each mixture into a dessert glass.

7. Layer the chopped nuts on top.

8. Cover the nuts with 1 tablespoon each of the chia mass.

9. Sprinkle the pomegranate seeds on top and serve everything.

**Nutrition:**

kcal: 248

Carbohydrates: 7 g

Protein: 1 g

Fat: 19 g

# Lavender Blueberry Chia Seed Pudding

**Prep Time:** 1 hour 10 minutes

**Cook Time:** 0 minutes

**Serves:** 4

**What you need:**

- 100 g blueberries

- 70 g organic quark

- 50 g soy yogurt

- 30 g hazelnuts

- 200 ml almond milk

- 2 tbsp chia seeds

- 2 teaspoons agave syrup

- 2 teaspoons of lavender

**Steps:**

1. Bring the almond milk to a boil along with the lavender.

2. Let the mixture simmer for 10 minutes at a reduced temperature.

3. Let them cool down afterwards.

4. If the milk is cold, add the blueberries and puree everything.

5. Mix the whole thing with the chia seeds and agave syrup.

6. Let everything soak in the refrigerator for an hour.

7. Mix the yogurt and curd cheese.

8. Add both to the crowd.

9. Divide the pudding into glasses.

10. Finely chop the hazelnuts and sprinkle them on top.

## Nutrition:

kcal: 252

Carbohydrates: 12 g

Protein: 1 g

Fat: 11 g

# Yogurt with Granola and Persimmon

**Prep Time:** 5 minutes

**Cook Time:** 5 minutes

**Serves:** 1

## What you need:

- 150g Greek style yogurt
- 20g oatmeal
- 60g fresh persimmons
- 30 ml of tap water

## Steps:

1. Put the oatmeal in the pan without any fat.

2. Toast them, stirring constantly, until golden brown.

3. Then put them on a plate and let them cool down briefly.

4. Peel the persimmon and put it in a bowl with the water. Mix the whole thing into a fine puree.

5. Put the yogurt, the toasted oatmeal, and the puree in layers in a glass and serve.

**Nutrition:**

kcal: 286

Carbohydrates: 29 g

Protein: 1 g

Fat: 11 g

# Smoothie Bowl with Spinach, Mango and Muesli

**Prep Time:** 10 minutes

**Cook Time:** 0 minutes

**Serves:** 1

**What you need:**

- 150g yogurt
- 30g apple
- 30g mango
- 30g low carb muesli
- 10g spinach
- 10g chia seeds

**Steps:**

1. Soak the spinach leaves and let them drain.

2. Peel the mango and cut it into strips.

3. Remove apple core and cut it into pieces.

4. Put everything except the mango together with the yogurt in a blender and make a fine puree out of it.

5. Put the spinach smoothie in a bowl.

6. Add the muesli, chia seeds, and mango.

7. Serve the whole thing

**Nutrition:**

kcal: 362

Carbohydrates: 21 g

Protein: 12 g

Fat: 21 g

# Fried Egg with Bacon

**Prep Time:** 5 minutes

**Cook Time:** 10 minutes

**Serves:** 1

**What you need:**

- 2 eggs
- 30 grams of bacon
- 2 tbsp olive oil
- salt
- pepper

**Steps:**

1. Heat oil in the pan and fry the bacon.

2. Reduce the heat and beat the eggs in the pan.

3. Cook the eggs and season with salt and pepper.

4. Serve the fried eggs hot with the bacon.

**Nutrition:**

kcal: 405

Carbohydrates: 1 g

Protein: 19 g

Fat: 38 g

# Smoothie Bowl with Berries, Poppy Seeds, Nuts and Seeds

**Prep Time:** 15 minutes

**Cook Time:** 0 minutes

**Serves:** 2

**What you need:**

- 5 chopped almonds
- 2 chopped walnuts
- 1 apple
- ¼ banana
- 300 g yogurt
- 60 g raspberries
- 20 g blueberries
- 20 g rolled oats, roasted in a pan
- 10 g poppy seeds
- 1 teaspoon pumpkin seeds
- Agave syrup

**Steps:**

1. Clean the fruit and let it drain.
2. Take some berries and set them aside.

3. Place the remaining berries in a tall mixing vessel.

4. Cut the banana into slices. Put a few aside.

5. Add the rest of the banana to the berries.

6. Remove the core of the apple and cut it into quarters.

7. Cut the quarters into thin wedges and set a few aside.

8. Add the remaining wedges to the berries.

9. Add the yogurt to the fruits and mix everything into a puree.

10. Sweeten the smoothie with the agave syrup.

11. Divide it into two bowls.

12. Serve it with the remaining fruit, poppy seeds, oatmeal, nuts and seeds.

**Nutrition:**

kcal: 284

Carbohydrates: 21 g

Protein: 11 g

Fat: 19 g

# Whole Grain Bread and Avocado

**Prep Time:** 5 minutes

**Cook Time:** 0 minutes

Serving: 1

**What you need:**

- 2 slices of whole meal bread
- 60 g of cottage cheese
- 1 stick of thyme
- ½ avocado

- ½ lime
- Chili flakes
- salt
- pepper

**Steps:**

1. Cut the avocado in half.
2. Remove the pulp and cut it into slices.
3. Pour the lime juice over it.
4. Wash the thyme and shake it dry.
5. Remove the leaves from the stem.
6. Brush the whole wheat bread with the cottage cheese.
7. Place the avocado slices on top.
8. Top with the chili flakes and thyme.
9. Add salt and pepper and serve.

**Nutrition:**

kcal: 490

Carbohydrates: 31 g

Protein: 19 g

Fat: 21 g

Tip: both frozen and fresh blueberries will work great in this recipe. The only difference will be that muffins using fresh blueberries will cook slightly quicker than those using frozen.

Nutrition:

Fat: 1 g

Carbohydrates: 45 g

Fiber: 2 g

Protein: 4 g

# Hemp Seed Porridge

Prep Time: 5 minutes

Cook Time: 5 minutes

Serves: 6

What you need:

- 3 cups cooked hemp seed
- 1 packet Stevia
- 1 cup coconut milk

Steps:

1. In a saucepan, mix the rice and the coconut milk over moderate heat for about 5 minutes as you stir it constantly.

2. Remove the pan from the burner then add the Stevia. Stir.

3. Serve in 6 bowls.

4. Enjoy.

Nutrition:

Calories: 236 kcal

Fat: 1.8 g

Carbs: 48.3 g

Protein: 7 g

# Walnut Crunch Banana Bread

Prep Time: 5 minutes

Cook Time: 1 hour and 30 minutes

Serves: 1

What you need:

- 4 ripe bananas
- 1/4 cup maple syrup
- 1 tablespoon apple cider vinegar
- 1 teaspoon vanilla extract
- 11/2 cups whole-wheat flour
- 1/2 teaspoon ground cinnamon
- 1/2 teaspoon baking soda
- 1/4 cup walnut pieces (optional)

Steps:

1. Preheat the oven to 350°F.
2. In a large bowl, use a fork or mixing spoon to mash the bananas until they reach a puréed consistency (small bits of banana are acceptable). Stir in the maple syrup, apple cider vinegar, and vanilla.
3. Stir in the flour, cinnamon, and baking soda. Fold in the walnut pieces (if using).
4. Gently pour the batter into a loaf pan, filling it no more than three-quarters of the way full. Bake for 1 hour, or until you can stick a knife into the middle and it comes out clean.
5. Remove from the oven and allow cooling on the countertop for a minimum of 30 minutes before serving.

Nutrition:

Fat: 1g

Carbohydrates: 40 g

Fiber: 5 g

Protein: 4 g

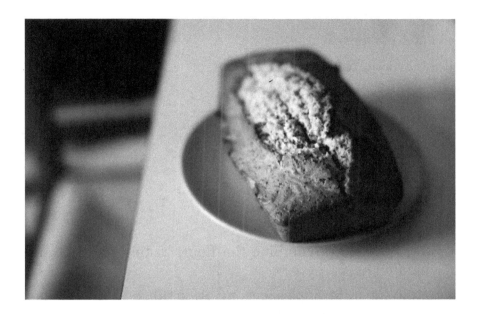

# Plant-Powered Pancakes

Prep Time: 5 minutes

Cook Time: 15 minutes

Serves: 8

What you need:

- 1 cup whole-wheat flour
- 1 teaspoon baking powder
- 1/2 teaspoon ground cinnamon
- 1 cup plant-based milk
- 1/2 cup unsweetened applesauce
- 1/4 cup maple syrup
- 1 teaspoon vanilla extract

Steps:

1. In a large bowl, combine the flour, baking powder, and cinnamon.
2. Stir in the milk, applesauce, maple syrup, and vanilla until no dry flour is left, and the batter is smooth.
3. Heat a large, nonstick skillet or griddle over medium heat. For each pancake, pour 1/4 cup of batter onto the hot skillet. Once bubbles form over the top of the pancake and the sides begin to brown, flip and cook for 1 or 2 minutes more.
4. Repeat until all of the batter is used, and serve.

Nutrition:

Fat: 2 g

Carbohydrates: 44 g

Fiber: 5 g

Protein: 5 g

# Mini Mac in a Bowl

Prep Time: 5 minutes

Cook Time: 15 minutes

Serves: 1

What you need:

- 5 ounces of lean ground beef
- Two tablespoons of diced white or yellow onion.
- 1/8 teaspoon of onion powder
- 1/8 teaspoon of white vinegar
- 1 ounce of dill pickle slices
- One teaspoon sesame seed
- 3 cups of shredded Romaine lettuce
- Cooking spray
- Two tablespoons reduced-fat shredded cheddar cheese
- Two tablespoons of Wish-Bone light thousand island as dressing

Steps:

1. Place a lightly greased small skillet on fire to heat.
2. Add your onion to cook for about 2-3 minutes.
3. Next, add the beef and allow cooking until it's brown.
4. Next, mix your vinegar and onion powder with the dressing.
5. Finally, top the lettuce with the cooked meat and sprinkle cheese on it, add your pickle slices.
6. Drizzle the mixture with the sauce and sprinkle the sesame seeds.
7. Your mini mac in a bowl is ready for consumption.

Nutrition:

Calories: 150

Protein: 21 g

Carbohydrates: 32 g

Fats: 19 g

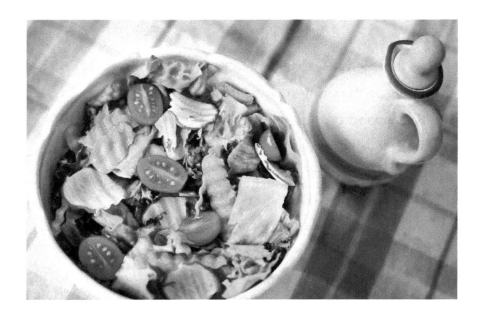

# Cake Fueling

Prep Time: 5 minutes

Cook Time: 0 minutes

Serves: 1

What you need:

- One packet of  shakes.

- 1/4 teaspoon of baking powder

- Two tablespoons of eggbeaters or egg whites

- Two tablespoons of water

- Other options that are not compulsory include sweetener, reduced-fat cream cheese, etc.

Steps:

1. Begin by preheating the oven.

2. Mix all the ingredients. Begin with the dry ingredients, and then add the wet ingredients.

3. After the mixture/batter is ready, pour gently into muffin cups.

4. Inside the oven, place, and bake for about 16-18 minutes or until it is baked and ready. Allow it to cool completely.

5. Add additional toppings of your choice and ensure your delicious shake cake is refreshing.

Nutrition:

Calories: 896

Fat: 37 g

Carbohydrate: 115 g

Protein: 34 g

# Biscuit Pizza

Prep Time: 5 minutes

Cook Time: 15-20 minutes

Serves: 1

What you need:

- 1/4 sachet of buttermilk cheddar and herb biscuit
- 1/4 tablespoon of tomato sauce
- 1/4 tablespoon of low-fat shredded cheese
- ¼ bottle of water
- Parchment paper

Steps:

1. Begin by preheating the oven to about 350°F
2. Mix the biscuit and water and stir properly.
3. In the parchment paper, pour the mixture and spread it into a thin circle. Allow cooking for 10 minutes.
4. Take it out and add the tomato sauce and shredded cheese.
5. Bake it for a few more minutes.

Nutrition:

Calories: 478

Protein: 30 g

Carbohydrates: 22 g

Fats: 29 g

# Lean and Green Smoothie 1

Prep Time: 5 minutes

Cook Time: 0 minutes

Serves: 1

What you need:

- 2 1/2 cups of kale leaves
- 3/4 cup of chilled apple juice
- 1 cup of cubed pineapple
- 1/2 cup of frozen green grapes
- 1/2 cup of chopped apple

Steps:

1. Place the pineapple, apple juice, apple, frozen seedless grapes, and kale leaves in a blender.
2. Cover and blend until it's smooth.
3. Smoothie is ready and can be garnished with halved grapes if you wish.

Nutrition:

Calories: 81

Protein: 2 g

Carbohydrates: 19 g

Fats: 1 g

# Lean and Green Smoothie 2

Prep Time: 5 minutes

Cook Time: 0 minutes

Serves: 1

What you need:

- Six kale leaves
- Two peeled oranges
- 2 cups of mango kombucha
- 2 cups of chopped pineapple
- 2 cups of water

Steps:

1. Break up the oranges, place in the blender.
2. Add the mango kombucha, chopped pineapple, and kale leaves into the blender.
3. Blend everything until it is smooth.
4. Smoothie is ready to be taken.

Nutrition:

Calories: 81

Protein: 2 g

Carbohydrates: 19 g

Fats: 1 g

# Lean and Green Chicken Pesto Pasta

Prep Time: 5 minutes

Cook Time: 15 minutes

Serves: 1

What you need:

- 3 cups of raw kale leaves
- 2 tbsp. of olive oil
- 2 cups of fresh basil
- 1/4 teaspoon salt
- 3 tbsp. lemon juice
- Three garlic cloves
- 2 cups of cooked chicken breast
- 1 cup of baby spinach
- 6 ounces of uncooked chicken pasta
- 3 ounces of diced fresh mozzarella
- Basil leaves or red pepper flakes to garnish

Steps:

1. Start by making the pesto; add the kale, lemon juice, basil, garlic cloves, olive oil, and salt to a blender and blend until it's smooth.

2. Add salt and pepper to taste.

3. Cook the pasta and strain off the water. Reserve 1/4 cup of the liquid.

4. Get a bowl and mix everything, the cooked pasta, pesto, diced chicken, spinach, mozzarella, and the reserved pasta liquid.

5. Sprinkle the mixture with additional chopped basil or red paper flakes (optional).

6. Now your salad is ready. You may serve it warm or chilled. Also, it can be taken as a salad mix-ins or as a side dish. Leftovers should be stored in the refrigerator inside an air-tight container for 3-5 days.

Nutrition:

Calories: 244

Protein: 20.5 g

Carbohydrates: 22.5 g

Fats: 10 g

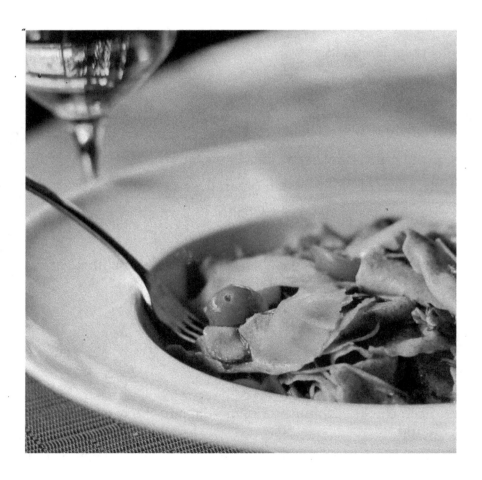

# Open-Face Egg Sandwiches with Cilantro-Jalapeño Spread

Prep Time: 20 minutes

Cook Time: 10 minutes

Serves: 2

What you need:

For the cilantro and jalapeño spread

- 1 cup filled up fresh cilantro leaves and stems (about a bunch)
- 1 jalapeño pepper, seeded and roughly chopped
- ½ cup extra-virgin olive oil
- ¼ cup pepitas (hulled pumpkin seeds), raw or roasted
- 2 garlic cloves, thinly sliced
- 1 tablespoon freshly squeezed lime juice
- 1 teaspoon kosher salt

For the eggs

- 4 large eggs
- ¼ cup milk
- ¼ to ½ teaspoon kosher salt
- 2 tablespoons butter

For the sandwich

- 2 slices bread
- 1 tablespoon butter
- 1 avocado, halved, pitted, and divided into slices
- Microgreens or sprouts, for garnish

Steps:

To make the cilantro and jalapeño spread

1. In a food processor, combine the cilantro, jalapeño, oil, pepitas, garlic, lime juice, and salt. Whirl until smooth. Refrigerate if making in advance; otherwise set aside.

To make the eggs

2. In a medium bowl, whisk the eggs, milk, and salt.

3. Dissolve the butter in a skillet over low heat, swirling to coat the bottom of the pan. Pour in the whisked eggs.

4. Cook until they begin to set then, using a heatproof spatula, push them to the sides, allowing the uncooked portions to run into the bottom of the skillet.

5. Continue until the eggs are set.

To assemble the sandwiches

1. Toast the bed and spread with butter.

2. Spread a spoonful of the cilantro-jalapeño spread on each piece of toast. Top each with scrambled eggs.

3. Arrange avocado over each sandwich and garnish with microgreens.

Nutrition:

Calories: 711

Total fat: 4 g

Cholesterol: 54 mg

Fiber: 12 g

Protein: 12 g

Sodium: 327 mg

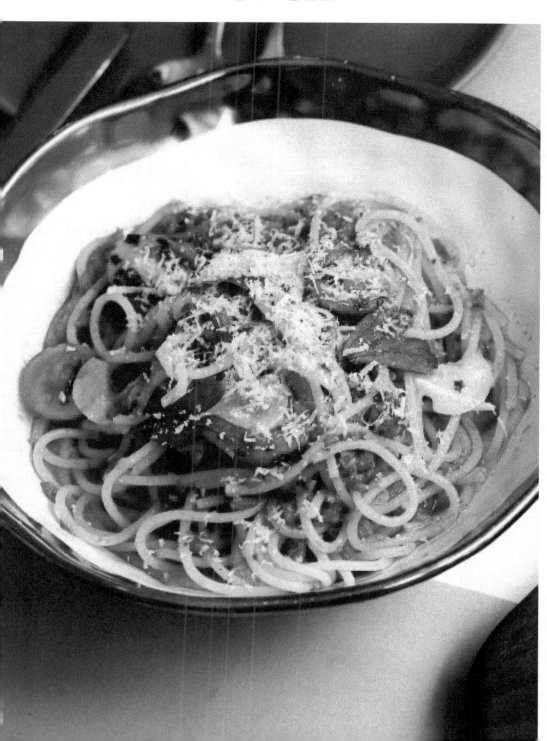

# Bacon Wrapped Asparagus

**Prep Time:** 10 minutes

**Cook Time:** 20 minutes

**Serves:** 2

**What you need:**

- 1/3 cup heavy whipping cream
- 2 bacon slices, precooked
- 4 small spears asparagus
- Salt, to taste
- 1 tablespoon butter

**Steps:**

1. Preheat the oven to 360 degrees and grease a baking sheet with butter.
2. Meanwhile, mix cream, asparagus and salt in a bowl.
3. Wrap the asparagus in bacon slices and arrange them in the baking dish.
4. Transfer the baking dish to the oven and bake for about 20 minutes.
5. Remove from the oven and serve hot.
6. Place the bacon wrapped asparagus in a dish and set aside to cool for meal prepping. Divide it in 2 containers and cover the lid. Refrigerate for about 2 days and reheat in the microwave before serving.

**Nutrition:**

Calories: 204
Carbs: 1.4g
Protein: 5.9g
Fat: 19.3g
Sugar: 0.5g

# Spinach Chicken

**Prep Time:** 10 minutes

**Cook Time:** 10 minutes

**Serves:** 2

**What you need:**

- 2 garlic cloves, minced
- 2 tablespoons unsalted butter, divided
- ¼ cup parmesan cheese, shredded
- ¾ pound chicken tenders
- ¼ cup heavy cream
- 10 ounces frozen spinach, chopped
- Salt and black pepper, to taste

**Steps:**

1. Heat 1 tablespoon of butter in a large skillet and add chicken, salt and black pepper.
2. Cook for about 3 minutes on both sides and remove the chicken to a bowl.
3. Melt remaining butter in the skillet and add garlic, cheese, heavy cream and spinach.
4. Cook for about 2 minutes and add the chicken.
5. Cook for about 5 minutes on low heat and dish out to immediately serve.
6. Place chicken in a dish and set aside to cool for meal prepping. Divide it in 2 containers and cover them. Refrigerate for about 3 days and reheat in microwave before serving.

**Nutrition:**

Calories: 288

Carbs: 3.6g

Protein: 27.7g

Fat: 18.3g

Sugar: 0.3g

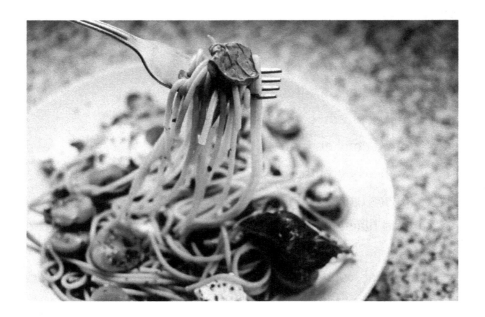

# Lemongrass Prawns

**Prep Time:** 10 minutes

**Cook Time:** 15 minutes

**Serves:** 2

**What you need:**

- ½ red chili pepper, seeded and chopped
- 2 lemongrass stalks
- ½ pound prawns, deveined and peeled
- 6 tablespoons butter
- ¼ teaspoon smoked paprika

**Steps:**

1. Preheat the oven to 390 degrees and grease a baking dish.
2. Mix red chili pepper, butter, smoked paprika and prawns in a bowl.
3. Marinate for about 2 hours and then thread the prawns on the lemongrass stalks.
4. Arrange the threaded prawns on the baking dish and transfer it in the oven.
5. Bake for about 15 minutes and dish out to serve immediately.
6. Place the prawns in a dish and set aside to cool for meal prepping. Divide it in 2 containers and close the lid. Refrigerate for about 4 days and reheat in microwave before serving.

**Nutrition:**

Calories: 322

Carbs: 3.8g

Protein: 34.8g

Fat: 18g

Sugar: 0.1g
Sodium: 478mg

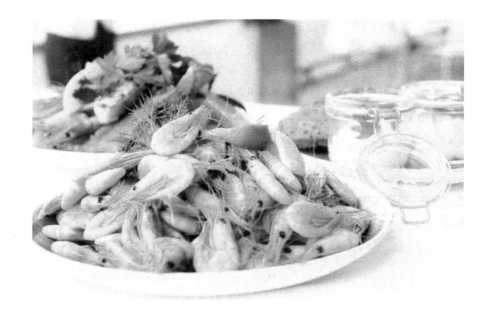

# Stuffed Mushrooms

**Prep Time:** 20 minutes

**Cook Time:** 25 minutes

**What you need:**

- 2 ounces bacon, crumbled
- ½ tablespoon butter
- ¼ teaspoon paprika powder
- 2 portobello mushrooms
- 1 oz cream cheese
- ¾ tablespoon fresh chives, chopped
- Salt and black pepper, to taste

**Steps:**

1. Preheat the oven to 400 degrees and grease a baking dish.
2. Heat butter in a skillet and add mushrooms.
3. Sauté for about 4 minutes and set aside.
4. Mix cream cheese, chives, paprika powder, salt and black pepper in a bowl.
5. Stuff the mushrooms with this mixture and transfer on the baking dish.
6. Place in the oven and bake for about 20 minutes.
7. These mushrooms can be refrigerated for about 3 days for meal prepping and can be served with scrambled eggs.

**Nutrition:**

Calories: 570

Carbs: 4.6g

Protein: 19.9g

Fat: 52.8g

Sugar: 0.8g

Sodium: 1041mg

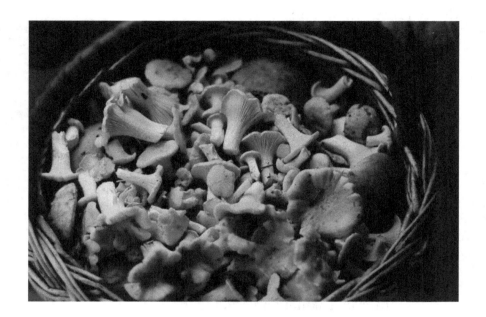

# Honey Glazed Chicken Drumsticks

**Prep Time:** 10 minutes

**Cook Time:** 20 minutes

**Serves:** 2

**What you need:**

- ½ tablespoon fresh thyme, minced
- 1/8 cup Dijon mustard
- ½ tablespoon fresh rosemary, minced
- ½ tablespoon honey
- 2 chicken drumsticks
- 1 tablespoon olive oil
- Salt and black pepper, to taste

**Steps:**

1. Preheat the oven at 325 degrees and grease a baking dish.
2. Combine all the ingredients in a bowl except the drumsticks and mix well.
3. Add drumsticks and coat generously with the mixture.
4. Cover and refrigerate to marinate overnight.
5. Place the drumsticks in in the baking dish and transfer it in the oven.
6. Cook for about 20 minutes and dish out to immediately serve.
7. Place chicken drumsticks in a dish and set aside to cool for meal prepping. Divide it in 2 containers and cover them. Refrigerate for about 3 days and reheat in microwave before serving.

**Nutrition:**

Calories: 301

Carbs: 6g

Fats: 19.7g

Proteins: 4.5g

Sugar: 4.5g

Sodium: 316mg

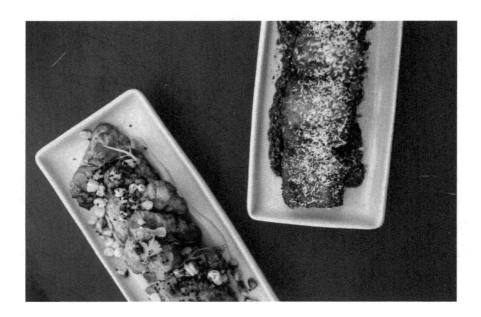

# Crab Cakes

**Prep Time:** 20 minutes

**Cook Time:** 10 minutes

**Serves:** 2

**What you need:**

- ½ pound lump crabmeat, drained
- 2 tablespoons coconut flour
- 1 tablespoon mayonnaise
- ¼ teaspoon green Tabasco sauce
- 3 tablespoons butter
- 1 small egg, beaten
- ¾ tablespoon fresh parsley, chopped
- ½ teaspoon yellow mustard
- Salt and black pepper, to taste

**Steps:**

1. Mix all the ingredients in a bowl except butter.
2. Make patties from this mixture and set aside.
3. Heat butter in a skillet over medium heat and add patties.
4. Cook for about 10 minutes on each side and dish out to serve hot.
5. You can store the raw patties in the freezer for about 3 weeks for meal prepping. Place patties in a container and place parchment paper in between the patties to avoid stickiness.

**Nutrition:**

Calories: 153

Fat: 10.8g

Carbs: 6.7g

Protein: 6.4g

Sugar: 2.4

Sodium: 46mg

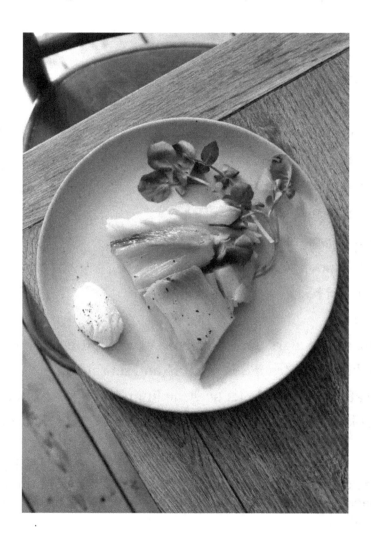

# Low Carb Black Beans Chili Chicken

**Prep Time:** 10 minutes

**Cook Time:** 25 minutes

**Serves:** 10

**What you need:**

- 1-3/4 pounds of chicken breasts, cubed (boneless skinless)
- 2 sweet red peppers, chopped
- 1 onion, chopped
- 3 tablespoons of olive oil
- 1 can of chopped green chiles
- 4 cloves of garlic, minced
- 2 tablespoons of chili powder
- 2 teaspoons of ground cumin
- 1 teaspoon of ground coriander
- 2 cans of black beans, rinsed and drained
- 1 can of Italian stewed tomatoes, cut up
- 1 cup of chicken broth or beer
- 1/2 to 1 cup of water

**Steps:**

1. Put oil into a skillet and place over medium heat. Add in the red pepper, chicken, and onion and cook until the chicken is brown, about five minutes.

2. Add in the garlic, chiles, chili powder, coriander, and cumin and cook for an additional minute.

3. Next, add in the tomatoes, beans, half cup of water, and broth and cook until it boils. Decrease the heat, uncover the skillet and cook while stirring for fifteen minutes.

4. Serve.

**Nutrition:**

Calories: 236

Fat: 6g

Protein: 22g

Carbohydrates: 21g

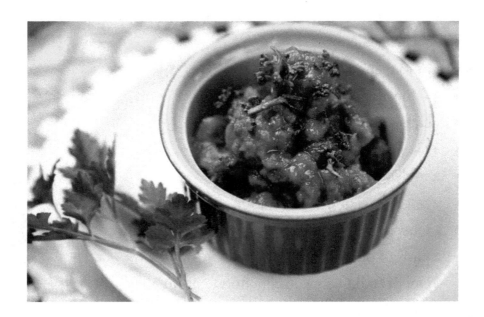

# Flavorful Taco Soup

**Prep Time:** 5 minutes

**Cook Time:** 15

**Serves:** 8

**What you need:**

- 1 lb of Ground beef
- 3 tablespoons of Taco seasoning, divided
- 4 cup of Beef bone broth
- 2 14.5-oz cans of Diced tomatoes
- 3/4 cup of Ranch dressing

**Steps:**

1. Put the ground beef into a pot and place over medium high heat and cook until brown, about ten minutes.
2. Add in ¾ cup of broth and two tablespoons of taco seasoning. Cook until part of the liquid has evaporated.
3. Add in the diced tomatoes, rest of the broth, and rest of the taco seasoning. Stir to mix, then simmer for ten minutes.
4. Remove the pot from heat, and add in the ranch dressing. Garnish with cilantro and cheddar cheese. Serve.

**Nutrition:**

Calories: 309

Fat: 24g

Protein: 13g

# Delicious Pot Buffalo Chicken Soup

**Prep Time:** 10 minutes

**Cook Time:** 20 minutes

**Serves:** 6

**What you need:**

- 1 tablespoon of Olive oil
- 1/2 Onion, diced)
- 1/2 cup of Celery, diced
- 4 cloves of Garlic, minced
- 1 lb of Shredded chicken, cooked
- 4 cup of Chicken bone broth, or any chicken broth
- 3 tablespoons of Buffalo sauce
- 6 oz of Cream cheese
- 1/2 cup of Half & half

**Steps:**

1. Switch the pot to the saute function. Add in the chopped onion, oil, and celery. Cook until the onions are brown and translucent, about ten minutes.

2. Add in the garlic and cook until fragrant, about one minute. Switch off the pot.

3. Add in the broth, shredded chicken, and buffalo sauce. Cover the pot and seal. Switch the soup feature on and set time to five minutes.

4. When cooked, release pressure naturally for five minutes and then quickly.

5. Scoop out one cup of the soup liquid into a blender bowl, then add in the cheese and blend until smooth. Pour the puree into the pot, then add in the calf and half and stir to mix.

6. Serve.

**Nutrition:**

**Serves:** 1 cup

Calories: 270

Protein: 27g

Fat: 16g

Carbohydrates: 4g

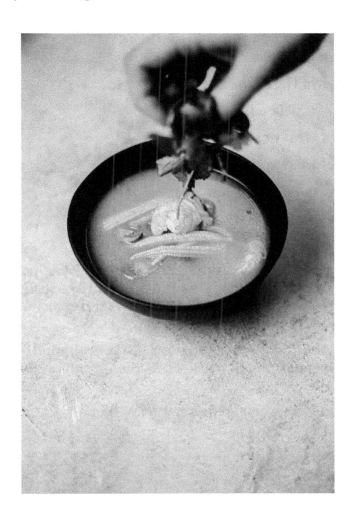

# Creamy Low Carb Cream of Mushroom Soup

**Prep Time:** 15 minutes

**Cook Time:** 15 minutes

**Serves:** 5

**What you need:**

- 1 tablespoons of Olive oil
- 1/2 Onion, diced
- 20 oz of Mushrooms, sliced
- 6 cloves of Garlic, minced
- 2 cup of Chicken broth
- 1 cup of Heavy cream
- 1 cup of Unsweetened almond milk
- 3/4 teaspoon of Sea salt
- 1/4 teaspoon of Black pepper

**Steps:**

1. Place a pot over medium heat and add in olive oil. Add in the mushrooms and onions and cook until browned, about fifteen minutes. Next, add in the garlic and cook for another one minute.

2. Add in the cream, chicken broth, sea salt, almond milk, and black pepper. Cook until boil, then simmer for fifteen minutes.

3. Puree the soup using an immersion blender until smooth. Serve.

**Nutrition:**

**Serves:** 1 cup

Calories: 229

Fat: 21g

Protein: 5g

Carbohydrates: 8g

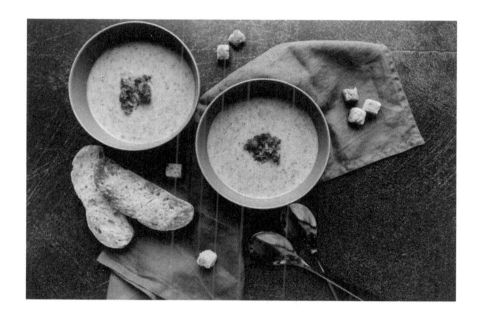

# Tropical Greens Smoothie

Prep Time: 5 Minutes

Cook Time: 0 Minutes

Serves: 1

What you need:

- One banana
- 1/2 large navel orange, peeled and segmented
- 1/2 cup frozen mango chunks
- 1 cup frozen spinach
- One celery stalk, broken into pieces
- One tablespoon cashew butter or almond butter
- 1/2 tablespoon spiraling
- 1/2 tablespoon ground flaxseed
- 1/2 cup unsweetened nondairy milk
- Water, for thinning (optional)

Steps:

1. In a high-speed blender or food processor, combine the bananas, orange, mango, spinach, celery, cashew butter, spiraling (if using), flaxseed, and milk.
2. Blend until creamy, adding more milk or water to thin the smoothie if too thick. Serve immediately—it is best served fresh.

Nutrition:

Calories: 391

Fat: 12g

Protein: 13g

Carbohydrates: 68g

Fiber: 13g

# Vitamin C Smoothie Cubes

Prep Time: 5 minutes

Cook Time: 8 hours to chill

Serves: 1

What you need:

- 1/8 large papaya
- 1/8 mango
- 1/4 cups chopped pineapple, fresh or frozen
- 1/8 cup raw cauliflower florets, fresh or frozen
- 1/4 large navel oranges, peeled and halved
- 1/4 large orange bell pepper stemmed, seeded, and coarsely chopped

Steps:

1. Halve the papaya and mango, remove the pits, and scoop their soft flesh into a high-speed blender.

2. Add the pineapple, cauliflower, oranges, and bell pepper. Blend until smooth.

3. Evenly divide the puree between 2 (16-compartment) ice cube trays and place them on a level surface in your freezer. Freeze for at least 8 hours.

4. The cubes can be left in the ice cube trays until use or transferred to a freezer bag. The frozen cubes are good for about three weeks in a standard freezer, or up to 6 months in a chest freezer.

Nutrition:

Calories: 96

Fat: 1 g

Protein: 2 g

Carbohydrates: 24 g

Fiber: 4 g

# Overnight Chocolate Chia Pudding

Prep Time: 2 minutes

Cook Time: overnight to chill

Serves: 1

What you need:

- 1/8 cup chia seeds
- 1/2 cup unsweetened nondairy milk
- One tablespoon raw cocoa powder
- 1/2 teaspoon vanilla extract
- 1/2 teaspoon pure maple syrup

Steps:

1. Stir together the chia seeds, milk, cacao powder, vanilla, and maple syrup in a large bowl.
2. Divide between two (1/2-pint) covered glass jars or containers.
3. Refrigerate overnight.
4. Stir before serving.

Nutrition:

Calories: 213

Fat: 10 g

Protein: 9 g

Carbohydrates: 20 g

Fiber: 15 g

# Slow Cooker Savory Butternut Squash Oatmeal

Prep Time: 15 minutes

Cook Time: 6 to 8 hours

Serves: 1

What you need:

- 1/4 cup steel-cut oats
- 1/2 cups cubed (1/2-inch pieces), peeled butternut squash (freeze any leftovers after preparing a whole squash for future meals)
- 3/4 cups of water
- 1/16 cup unsweetened nondairy milk
- 1/4 tablespoon chia seeds
- 1/2 teaspoons yellow miso paste
- 3/4 teaspoons ground ginger
- 1/4 tablespoon sesame seeds, toasted
- 1/4 tablespoon chopped scallion, green parts only
- Shredded carrot, for serving (optional)

Steps:

1. In a slow cooker, combine the oats, butternut squash, and water.

2. Cover the slow cooker and cook on low for 6 to 8 hours, or until the squash is fork-tender.

3. Using a potato masher or heavy spoon, roughly mash the cooked butternut squash.

4. Stir to combine with the oats.

5. Whisk together the milk, chia seeds, miso paste, and ginger in a large bowl. Stir the mixture into the oats.

6. Top your oatmeal bowl with sesame seeds and scallion for more plant-based fiber, top with shredded carrot (if using).

Nutrition:

Calories: 230

Fat: 5 g

Protein: 7 g

Carbohydrates: 40 g

Fiber: 9 g

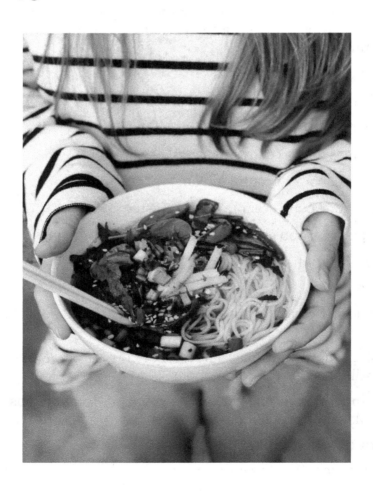

# Carrot Cake Oatmeal

Prep Time: 10 minutes

Cook Time: 15 minutes

Serves: 1

What you need:

- 1/8 cup pecans
- 1/2 cup finely shredded carrot
- 1/4 cup old-fashioned oats
- 5/8 cups unsweetened nondairy milk
- 1/2 tablespoon pure maple syrup
- 1/2 teaspoon ground cinnamon
- 1/2 teaspoon ground ginger
- 1/8 teaspoon ground nutmeg
- One tablespoon chia seed

Steps:

1. Over medium-high heat in a skillet, toast the pecans for 3 to 4 minutes, often stirring, until browned and fragrant (watch closely, as they can burn quickly).
2. Pour the pecans onto a cutting board and coarsely chop them. Set aside.
3. In an 8-quart pot over medium-high heat, combine the carrot, oats, milk, maple syrup, cinnamon, ginger, and nutmeg.
4. When it is already boiling, reduce the heat to medium-low.
5. Cook, uncovered, for 10 minutes, stirring occasionally.
6. Stir in the chopped pecans and chia seeds. Serve immediately.

Nutrition:

Calories: 307

Fat: 17 g

Protein: 7 g

Carbohydrates: 35 g

Fiber: 11 g

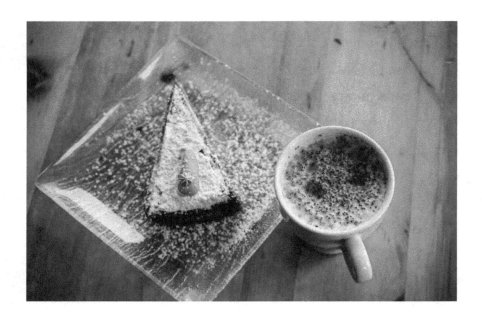

# Bacon Spaghetti Squash Carbonara

Prep Time: 20 minutes

Cook Time: 40 minutes

Serves: 4

What you need:

- 1 small spaghetti squash
- 6 ounces' bacon (roughly chopped)
- 1 large tomato (sliced)
- 2 chives (chopped)
- 1 garlic clove (minced)
- 6 ounces low-fat cottage cheese
- 1 cup Gouda cheese (grated)
- 2 tablespoons olive oil
- Salt and pepper, to taste

Steps:

1. Preheat the oven to 350°F.

2. Cut the squash spaghetti in half, brush with some olive oil and bake for 20–30 minutes, skin side up. Remove from the oven and remove the core with a fork, creating the spaghetti.

3. Heat one tablespoon of olive oil in a skillet. Cook the bacon for about 1 minute until crispy.

4. Quickly wipe out the pan with paper towels.

5. Heat another tablespoon of oil and sauté the garlic, tomato, and chives for 2–3 minutes. Add the spaghetti and sauté for another 5 minutes, occasionally stirring to keep from burning.

6. Begin to add the cottage cheese, about two tablespoons at a time. If the sauce becomes thick, add about a cup of water.

The sauce should be creamy but not too runny or thick. Allow cooking for another 3 minutes.

7. Serve immediately.

Nutrition:

Calories: 305

Total Fat: 21 g

Net Carbs: 8 g

Protein: 18 g

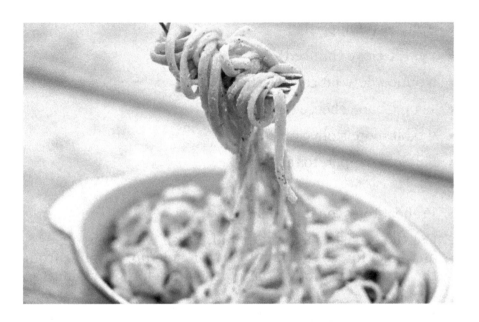

# Spiced Sorghum and Berries

Prep Time: 5 minutes

Cook Time: 1 hour

Serves: 1

What you need:

- 1/4 cup whole-grain sorghum
- 1/4 teaspoon ground cinnamon
- 1/4 teaspoon Chinese five-spice powder
- 3/4 cups water
- 1/4 cup unsweetened nondairy milk
- 1/4 teaspoon vanilla extract
- 1/2 tablespoons pure maple syrup
- 1/2 tablespoon chia seed
- 1/8 cup sliced almonds
- 1/2 cups fresh raspberries, divided

Steps:

1. Using a large pot over medium-high heat, stir together the sorghum, cinnamon, five-spice powder, and water.

2. Wait for the water to a boil, cover it, and reduce the heat to medium-low.

3. Cook for one hour, or until the sorghum is soft and chewy. If the sorghum grains are still hard, add another water cup and cook for 15 minutes more.

4. Using a glass measuring cup, whisk together the milk, vanilla, and maple syrup to blend.

5. Add the mixture to the sorghum and the chia seeds, almonds, and one cup of raspberries. Gently stir to combine.

6. When serving, top with the remaining one cup of fresh raspberries.

Nutrition:

Calories: 289

Fat: 8 g

Protein: 9 g

Carbohydrates: 52 g

Fiber: 10 g

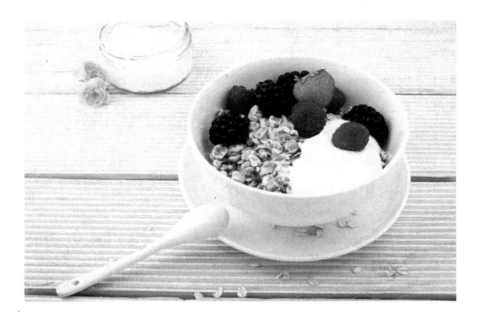

# Raw-Cinnamon-Apple Nut Bowl

Prep Time: 15 minutes

Cook Time: 1 hour to chill

Serves: 1

What you need:

- One green apple halved, seeded, and cored
- 3/4 Honeycrisp apples, halved, seeded, and cored
- 1/4 teaspoon freshly squeezed lemon juice
- One pitted Medrol dates
- 1/8 teaspoon ground cinnamon
- Pinch ground nutmeg
- 1/2 tablespoons chia seeds, plus more for serving (optional)
- 1/4 tablespoon hemp seed
- 1/8 cup chopped walnuts
- Nut butter, for serving (optional)

Steps:

1. Finely dice half the green apple and one Honey crisp apple. With the lemon juice, store it in an airtight container while you work on the next steps.

2. Coarsely chop the remaining apples and the dates. Transfer to a food processor and add the cinnamon and nutmeg.

3. Check it several times to see if it's mixing, then processes for 2 to 3 minutes to puree. Stir the puree into the reserved diced apples.

4. Stir in the chia seeds (if using), hemp seeds, and walnuts.

5. Chill for at least one hour.

6. Enjoy!

7. Serve as it is or top with additional chia seeds and nut butter (if using).

Nutrition:

Calories: 274

Fat: 8 g

Protein: 4 g

Carbohydrates: 52 g

Fiber: 9 g

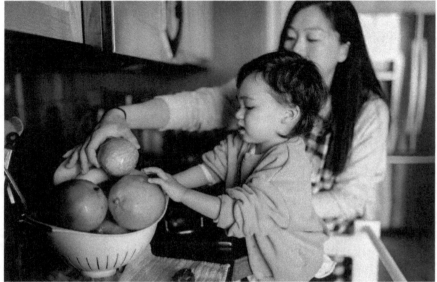

# DINNER

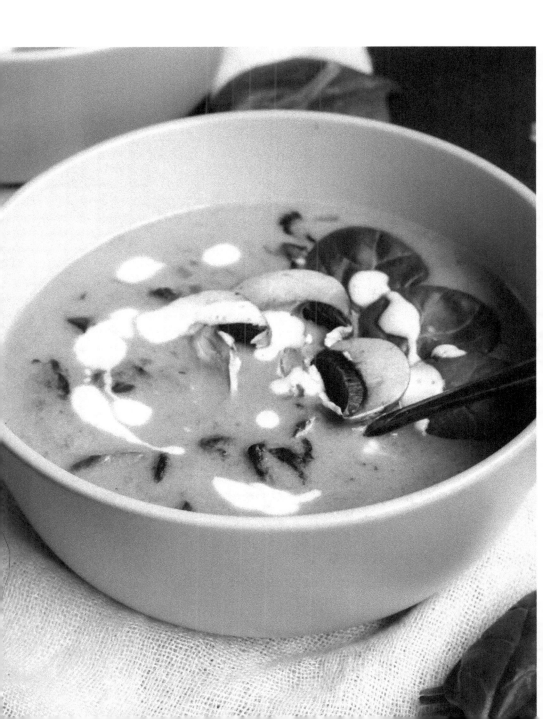

# Red Quinoa and Black Bean Soup

**Prep Time:** 5 minutes

**Cook Time:** 40 minutes

**Serves:** 6

**What you need:**

- 1 1/4 cup red quinoa
- 4 minced garlic cloves
- 1/2 tablespoon coconut oil
- 1 diced jalapeno
- 3 cups diced onion
- 2 teaspoon cumin
- 1 chopped sweet potato
- 1 teaspoon coriander
- 1 teaspoon chili powder
- 5 cups vegetable broth
- 15 ounces black beans
- 1/2 teaspoon cayenne pepper
- 2 cups spinach

**Steps:**

1. Begin by bringing the quinoa into a saucepan to boil with two cups of water. Allow the quinoa to simmer for twenty minutes. Next, remove the quinoa from the heat.

2. To the side, heat the oil, the onion, and the garlic together in a large soup pot.

3. Add the jalapeno and the sweet potato and sauté for an additional seven minutes.

4. Next, add all the spices and the broth and bring the soup to a simmer for twenty-five minutes. The potatoes should be soft.

5. Prior to serving, add the quinoa, the black beans, and the spinach to the mix. Season, and serve warm. Enjoy.

Nutrition:

Calories: 211

Carbs: 22g

Fat: 7g

Protein: 19g

# October Potato Soup

**Prep Time:** 5 minutes

**Cook Time:** 20 minutes

**Serves:** 3

**What you need:**

- 4 minced garlic cloves
- 2 teaspoon coconut oil
- 3 diced celery stalks
- 1 diced onion
- 2 teaspoon yellow mustard seeds
- 5 diced Yukon potatoes
- 6 cups vegetable broth
- 1 teaspoon oregano
- 1 teaspoon paprika
- 1/2 teaspoon cayenne pepper
- 1 teaspoon chili powder
- Salt and pepper to taste

**Steps:**

1. Begin by sautéing the garlic and the mustard seeds together in the oil in a large soup pot.

2. Next, add the onion and sauté the mixture for another five minutes.

3. Add the celery, the broth, the potatoes, and all the spices, and continue to stir.

4. Allow the soup to simmer for thirty minutes without a cover.

5. Next, Position about three cups of the soup in a blender, and puree the soup until you've reached a smooth

consistency. Pour this back into the big soup pot, stir, and serve warm. Enjoy.

Nutrition:

Calories: 203

Carbs: 12g

Fat: 7g

Protein: 9g

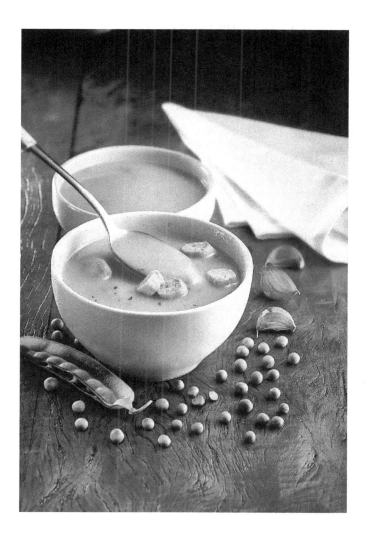

# Chicken Relleno Casserole

**Prep Time:** 19 minutes

**Cook Time:** 29 minutes

**Serves:** 6

**What you need:**

- 6 Tortilla Factory low-carb whole wheat tortillas, torn into small pieces
- 1 ½ cups hand-shredded cheese, Mexican
- 1 beaten egg
- 1 cup milk
- 2 cups cooked chicken, shredded
- 1 can Ro-tel
- ½ cup salsa verde

**Steps:**

1. Grease an 8 x 8 glass baking dish
2. Heat oven to 375 degrees
3. Combine everything together, but reserve ½ cup of the cheese
4. Bake it for 29 minutes
5. Take it out of oven and add ½ cup cheese
6. Broil for about 2 minutes to melt the cheese

**Nutrition:**

Calories: 265

Total Fat: 16g

Protein: 20g

Total Carbs: 18g

Dietary Fiber: 10g

Sugar: 0g
Sodium: 708mg

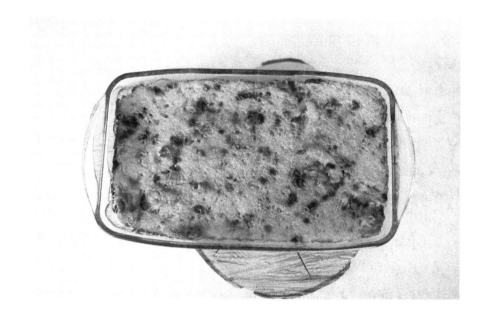

# Italian Chicken with Asparagus and Artichoke Hearts

**Prep Time:** 9 minutes

**Cook Time:** 40 minutes

**Serves:** 1

**What you need:**

- 1 can long asparagus spears, drained
- 1 c red peppers, roasted, drained
- 1 c artichoke hearts, drained
- 6 oz. of boneless chicken breast, pounded thin or sliced thinly
- 2 T parmesan cheese
- 1 T Bisquick
- ½ teaspoon oregano
- ½ teaspoon garlic powder
- ½ cup fresh sliced mushrooms
- 2 T red wine vinegar
- 2 T butter
- 3 T olive oil

**Steps:**

1. Place in a small blender container (or bowl) the oregano, garlic powder, vinegar, and 1 T oil. Place to the side.
2. Combine the Bisquick and Parmesan cheese.
3. Roll the chicken in the Bisquick and Parmesan mix.
4. Heat the butter in a skillet.
5. Brown the chicken on both sides and cook until done, approximately 4 minutes.

6. Emulsify or quickly whip the wet ingredients you have placed to the side. This is your dressing.

7. Place the chicken on the plate.

8. Surround with the vegetables and drizzle them with the dressing.

**Nutrition:**

Calories: 435

Total Fat: 18g

Protein: 38g

Total Carbs: 16g

Dietary Fiber: 7g

Sugar: 1g

Sodium: 860mg

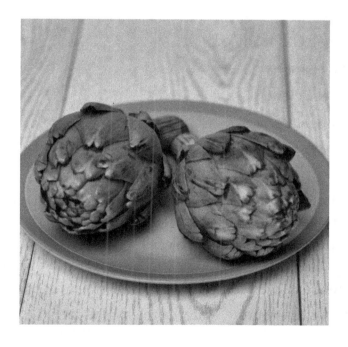

# Kabobs with Peanut Curry Sauce

**Prep Time:** 9 minutes

**Cook Time:** 9 minutes

**Serves:** 4

**What you need:**

- 1 cup Cream
- 4 teaspoon Curry Powder
- 1 1/2 teaspoon Cumin
- 1 1/2 teaspoon Salt
- 1 T minced garlic
- 1/3 cup Peanut Butter, sugar-free
- 2 T Lime Juice
- 3 T Water
- 1/2 small Onion, diced
- 2 T Soy Sauce
- 1 packet Splenda
- 8 oz. boneless, cooked Chicken Breast
- 8 oz. pork tenderloin

**Steps:**

1. Blend together cream, onion, 2 teaspoon. garlic, curry and cumin powder, and salt.

2. Slice the meats into 1 inch pieces.

3. Place the cream sauce into a bowl and put in the chicken and tenderloin to marinate. Let rest in sauce for 14 minutes.

4. Blend peanut butter, water, 1 teaspoon. garlic, lime juice, soy sauce, and Splenda. This is your peanut dipping sauce.

5. Remove the meats and thread on skewers. Broil or grill 4 minutes per side until meat is done.

6. Serve with dipping sauce.

**Nutrition:**

Calories: 530

Total Fat: 29g

Protein: 37g

Total Carbs: 6g

Dietary Fiber: 4g

Sugar: 2g

Sodium: 1538mg

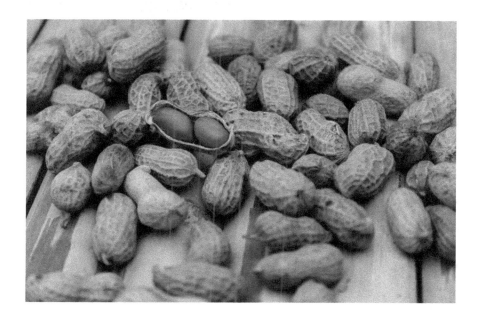

# Pizza

**Prep Time:** 4 minutes

**Cook Time:** 4 minutes

**Serves:** 1

**What you need:**

- 1 Tortilla Factory low carb whole wheat tortilla
- ¼ cup mozzarella cheese, hand-shredded
- ¼ cup tomato paste
- sprinkle of Italian seasoning
- sprinkle of garlic salt
- Cut the broccoli, spinach, mushrooms, peppers, and onions you like for toppings

**Steps:**

1. Turn broiler on in oven, or toaster oven
2. Spread tortilla with tomato paste
3. Sprinkle seasoning on the paste
4. Add the cheese
5. Add the veggies
6. Broil or toast 1-4 minutes until crust is crunchy and cheese melted

**Nutrition:**
Calories: 155
Total Fat: 7g
Protein: 13g
Total Carbs: 18g
Dietary Fiber: 10g
Sugar: 2g
Sodium: 741mg

# Salmon with Bok-Choy

**Prep Time:** 9 minutes

**Cook Time:** 9 minutes

**Serves:** 4

**What you need:**

- 1 c red peppers, roasted, drained
- 2 cups chopped bok-choy
- 1 T salted butter
- 5 oz. salmon steak
- 1 lemon, sliced very thinly
- 1/8 teaspoon black pepper
- 1 T olive oil
- 2 T sriracha sauce

**Steps:**

1. Place oil in skillet
2. Place all but 4 slices of lemon in the skillet.
3. Sprinkle the bok choy with the black pepper.
4. Stir fry the bok-choy with the lemons.
5. Remove and place on four plates.
6. Place the butter in the skillet and stir fry the salmon, turning once.
7. Place the salmon on the bed of bok-choy.
8. Divide the red peppers and encircle the salmon.
9. Place a slice of lemon atop the salmon.
10. Drizzle with sriracha sauce.

**Nutrition:**

Calories: 410

Total Fat: 30g

Protein: 30g

Total Carbs: 7g

Dietary Fiber: 2g

Sugar: 0g

Sodium: 200mg

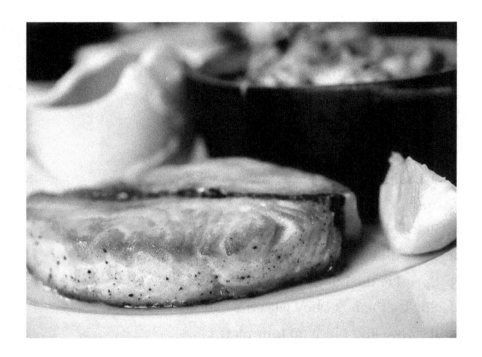

# Sriracha Tuna Kabobs

**Prep Time:** 4 minutes

**Cook Time:** 9 minutes

**Serves:** 4

**What you need:**

- 4 T Huy Fong chili garlic sauce
- 1 T sesame oil infused with garlic
- 1 T ginger, fresh, grated
- 1 T garlic, minced
- 1 red onion, cut into quarters and separated by petals
- 2 cups bell peppers, red, green, yellow
- 1 can whole water chestnuts, cut in half
- ½ pound fresh mushrooms, halved
- 32 oz. boneless tuna, chunks or steaks
- 1 Splenda packet
- 2 zucchini, sliced 1 inch thick, keep skins on

**Steps:**

1. Layer the tuna and the vegetable pieces evenly onto 8 skewers.
2. Combine the spices and the oil and chili sauce, add the Splenda
3. Quickly blend, either in blender or by quickly whipping.
4. Brush onto the kabob pieces, make sure every piece is coated
5. Grill 4 minutes on each side, check to ensure the tuna is cooked to taste.
6. Serving size is two skewers.

**Nutrition:**

Calories: 467
Total Fat: 18g
Protein: 56g
Total Carbs: 21g
Dietary Fiber: 3.5g
Sugar: 6g
Sodium: 433mg

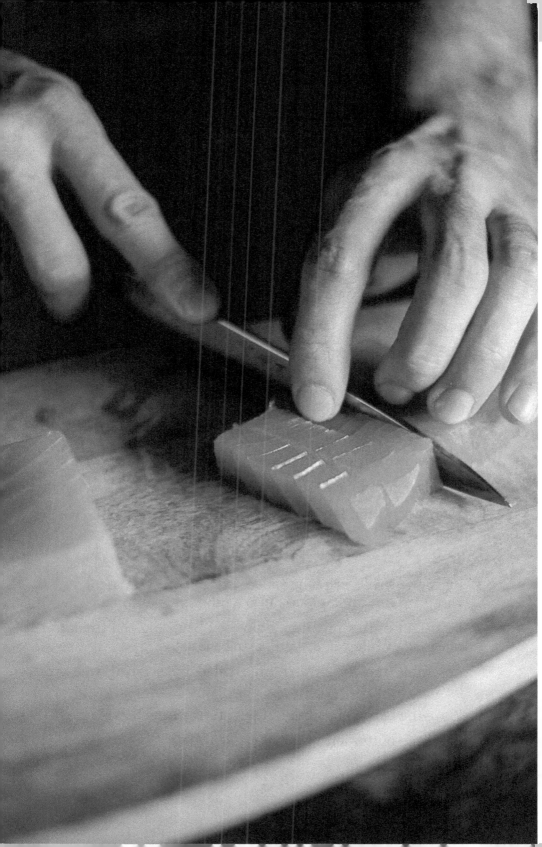

# Steak Salad with Asian Spice

**Prep Time:** 4 minutes

**Cook Time:** 4 minutes

**Serves:** 2

**What you need:**

- 2 T sriracha sauce
- 1 T garlic, minced
- 1 T ginger, fresh, grated
- 1 bell pepper, yellow, cut in thin strips
- 1 bell pepper, red, cut in thin strips
- 1 T sesame oil, garlic
- 1 Splenda packet
- ½ teaspoon curry powder
- ½ teaspoon rice wine vinegar
- 8 oz. of beef sirloin, cut into strips
- 2 cups baby spinach, stemmed
- ½ head butter lettuce, torn or chopped into bite-sized pieces

**Steps:**

1. Place the garlic, sriracha sauce, 1 teaspoon sesame oil, rice wine vinegar, and Splenda into a bowl and combine well.

2. Pour half of this mix into a zip-lock bag. Add the steak to marinade while you are preparing the salad.

3. Assemble the brightly colored salad by layering in two bowls.

4. Place the baby spinach into the bottom of the bowl.

5. Place the butter lettuce next.

6. Mix the two peppers and place on top.

7. Remove the steak from the marinade and discard the liquid and bag.

8. Heat the sesame oil and quickly stir fry the steak until desired doneness, it should take about 3 minutes.

9. Place the steak on top of the salad.

10.    Drizzle with the remaining dressing (other half of marinade mix).

11. Sprinkle sriracha sauce across the salad.

## Nutrition:

Calories: 350

Total Fat: 23g

Protein: 28g

Total Carbs: 7g

Dietary Fiber: 3.5

Sugar: 0

Sodium: 267mg

# Tilapia and Broccoli

**Prep Time:** 4 minutes

**Cook Time:** 14 minutes

**Serves:** 1

**What you need:**

- 6 oz. tilapia, frozen is fine

- 1 T butter

- 1 T garlic, minced or finely chopped

- 1 teaspoon of lemon pepper seasoning

- 1 cup broccoli florets, fresh or frozen, but fresh will be crisper

**Steps:**

1. Set the pre-warmed oven for 350 degrees.
2. Place the fish in an aluminum foil packet.
3. Arrange the broccoli around the fish to make an attractive arrangement.
4. Sprinkle the lemon pepper on the fish.
5. Close the packet and seal, bake for 14 minutes.
6. Combine the garlic and butter. Set aside.
7. Remove the packet from the oven and transfer ingredients to a plate.
8. Place the butter on the fish and broccoli.

**Nutrition:**

Calories: 362

Total Fat: 25g

Protein: 29g

Total Carbs: 3.5g

Dietary Fiber: 3g

Sugar: 0g

Sodium: 0mg

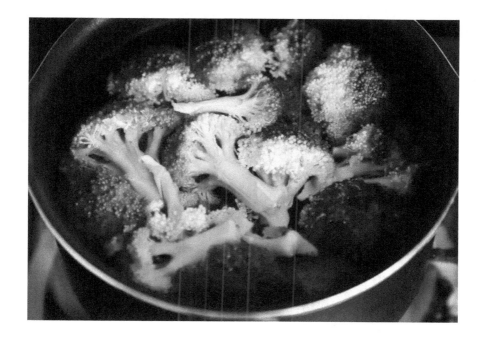

# Brown Basmati Rice Pilaf

Prep Time: 10 minutes

Cook Time: 3 minutes

Serves: 2

What you need:

- ½ tablespoon vegan butter
- ½ cup mushrooms, chopped
- ½ cup brown basmati rice
- 2-3 tablespoons water
- 1/8 teaspoon dried thyme
- Ground pepper to taste
- ½ tablespoon olive oil
- ¼ cup green onion, chopped
- 1 cup vegetable broth
- ¼ teaspoon salt
- ¼ cup chopped, toasted pecans

Steps:

1. Place a saucepan over medium-low heat. Add butter and oil.
2. When it melts, add mushrooms and cook until slightly tender.
3. Stir in the green onion and brown rice. Cook for 3 minutes. Stir constantly.
4. Stir in the broth, water, salt, and thyme.
5. When it begins to boil, lower the heat and cover with a lid. Simmer until rice is cooked. Add more water or broth if required.
6. Stir in the pecans and pepper.

7. Serve.

Nutrition:

Calories 189

Fats 11 g

Carbohydrates 19 g

Proteins 4 g

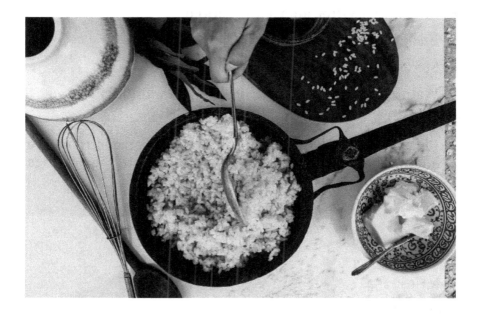

# Walnut and Date Porridge

Prep Time: 10 minutes

Cook Time: 0 minutes

Serves: 1

What you need:

- Strawberries, ½ cup (hulled)
- Milk or dairy-free alternative, 200 ml
- Buckwheat flakes, ½ cup
- Medjool date, 1 (chopped)
- Walnut butter, 1 teaspoon, or chopped walnut halves

Steps:

1. Place the date and the milk in a pan, heat gently before adding the buckwheat flakes. Then cook until the porridge gets to your desired consistency.

2. Add the walnuts, stir, then top with the strawberries.

3. Serve.

Nutrition:

Calories: 254

Protein: 65 g

Fat: 4 g

Vitamin B

# Vietnamese Turmeric Fish with Mango and Herbs Sauce

Prep Time: 15 minutes

Cook Time: 30 minutes

Serves: 4

What you need:

For the Fish:

- Coconut oil to fry the fish, 2 tablespoons
- Fresh codfish, skinless and boneless, 1 ¼ lbs. (cut into 2-inch piece wide)
- Pinch of sea salt, to taste

Fish Marinade:

- Chinese cooking wine, 1 tablespoon
- Turmeric powder, 1 tablespoon
- Sea salt, 1 teaspoon
- Olive oil, 2 tablespoons
- Minced ginger, 2 teaspoons

Mango Dipping Sauce:

- Juice of ½ lime
- Medium-sized ripe mango, 1
- Rice vinegar, 2 tablespoons
- Dry red chili pepper, 1 teaspoon (stir in before serving)
- Garlic clove, 1
- Infused scallion and dill oil
- Fresh dill, 2 cups
- Scallions, 2 cups (slice into long thin shape)

- A pinch of sea salt, to taste.

Toppings

- Nuts (pine or cashew nuts)
- Lime juice (as much as you like)
- Fresh cilantro (as much as you like)

Steps:

1. Add all the ingredients under "Mango Dipping Sauce" into your food processor. Blend until you get your preferred consistency.

2. Add two tablespoons of coconut oil in a large non-stick frying pan and heat over high heat. Once hot, add the pre-marinated fish. Add the slices of the fish into the pan individually. Divide into batches for easy frying, if necessary.

3. Once you hear a loud sizzle, reduce the heat to medium-high.

4. Do not move or turn the fish until it turns golden brown on one side; then turn it to the other side to fry, about 5 minutes on each side. Add more coconut oil to the pan if needed. Season with the sea salt.

5. Transfer the fish to a large plate. You will have some oil left in the frypan, which you will use to make your scallion and dill infused oil.

6. Using the remaining oil in the frypan, set to medium-high heat, add 2 cups of dill, and 2 cups of scallions.

7. Put off the heat after you have added the dill and scallions. Toss them gently for about 15 seconds, until the dill and scallions have wilted. Add a dash of sea salt to season.

8. Pour the dill, scallion, and infused oil over the fish. Serve with mango dipping sauce, nuts, lime, and fresh cilantro.

Nutrition:

Calories: 234

Fat: 23 g

Protein: 76 g

Sugar: 5 g

# Chicken and Kale Curry

Prep Time: 20 min

Cook Time: 1 hour

Serves: 3

What you need:

- Boiling water, 250 ml
- Skinless and boneless chicken thighs, 7 oz.
- Ground turmeric, 2 tablespoons
- Olive oil, 1 tablespoon
- Red onions, 1 (diced)
- Bird's eye chili, 1 (finely chopped)
- Freshly chopped ginger, ½ tablespoon
- Curry powder, ½ tablespoon
- Garlic, 1 ½ cloves (crushed)
- Cardamom pods, 1
- Tinned coconut milk, light, 100 ml
- Chicken stock, 2 cups
- Tinned chopped tomatoes, 1 cup

Direction:

1. Place the chicken thighs in a non-metallic bowl, add one tablespoon of turmeric and one teaspoon of olive oil. Mix together and keep aside to marinate for approx. 30 minutes.

2. Fry the chicken thighs over medium heat for about 5 minutes until well cooked and brown on all sides. Remove from the pan and set aside.

3. Add the remaining oil into a frypan on medium heat. Then add the onion, ginger, garlic, and chili. Fry for about 10 minutes until soft.

4. Add one tablespoon of the turmeric and half a tablespoon of curry powder to the pan and cook for another 2 minutes.

5. Then add the cardamom pods, coconut milk, tomatoes, and chicken stock. Allow simmering for thirty minutes.

6. Add the chicken once the sauce has reduced a little into the pan, followed by the kale. Cook until the kale is tender and the chicken is warm enough.

7. Serve with buckwheat.

8. Garnish with the chopped coriander.

Nutrition:

Calories: 313 g

Protein: 13 g

Fat: 6 g

Carbohydrate: 23 g

## VOLUME EQUIVALENTS(DRY)

| US STANDARD | METRIC (APPROXIMATE) |
|---|---|
| 1/8 teaspoon | 0.5 mL |
| 1/4 teaspoon | 1 mL |
| 1/2 teaspoon | 2 mL |
| 3/4 teaspoon | 4 mL |
| 1 teaspoon | 5 mL |
| 1 tablespoon | 15 mL |
| 1/4 cup | 59 mL |
| 1/2 cup | 118 mL |
| 3/4 cup | 177 mL |
| 1 cup | 235 mL |
| 2 cups | 475 mL |
| 3 cups | 700 mL |
| 4 cups | 1 L |

## VOLUME EQUIVALENTS(LIQUID)

| US STANDARD | US STANDARD (OUNCES) | METRIC (APPROXIMATE) |
|---|---|---|
| 2 tablespoons | 1 fl.oz. | 30 mL |
| 1/4 cup | 2 fl.oz. | 60 mL |
| 1/2 cup | 4 fl.oz. | 120 mL |
| 1 cup | 8 fl.oz. | 240 mL |
| 1 1/2 cup | 12 fl.oz. | 355 mL |
| 2 cups or 1 pint | 16 fl.oz. | 475 mL |
| 4 cups or 1 quart | 32 fl.oz. | 1 L |
| 1 gallon | 128 fl.oz. | 4 L |

## TEMPERATURES EQUIVALENTS

| FAHRENHEIT(F) | CELSIUS(C) (APPROXIMATE) |
|---|---|
| 225 °F | 107 °C |
| 250 °F | 120 °C |
| 275 °F | 135 °C |
| 300 °F | 150 °C |
| 325 °F | 160 °C |
| 350 °F | 180 °C |
| 375 °F | 190 °C |
| 400 °F | 205 °C |
| 425 °F | 220 °C |
| 450 °F | 235 °C |
| 475 °F | 245 °C |
| 500 °F | 260 °C |

## WEIGHT EQUIVALENTS

| US STANDARD | METRIC (APPROXIMATE) |
|---|---|
| 1 ounce | 28 g |
| 2 ounces | 57 g |
| 5 ounces | 142 g |
| 10 ounces | 284 g |
| 15 ounces | 425 g |
| 16 ounces (1 pound) | 455 g |
| 1.5 pounds | 680 g |
| 2 pounds | 907 g |

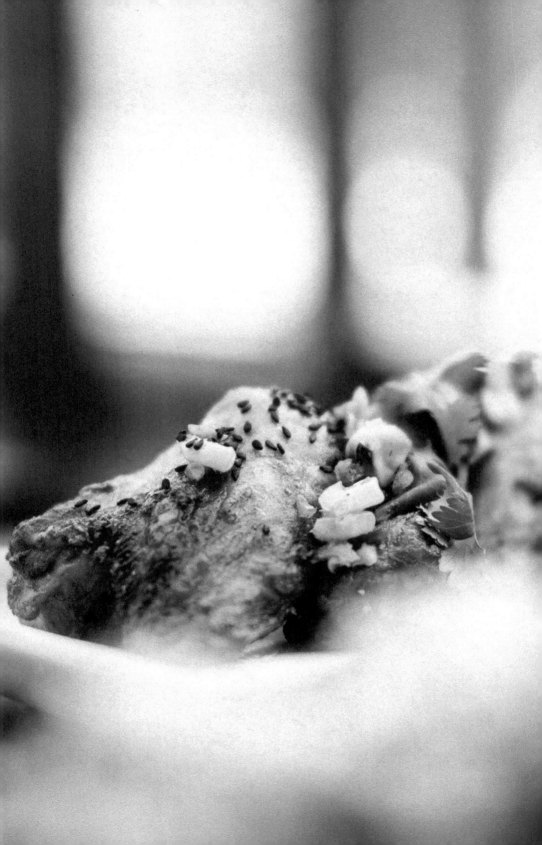

CPSIA information can be obtained
at www.ICGtesting.com
Printed in the USA
BVHW090724230621
610212BV00009B/1316

# The Ultimate Intermittent Fasting Cookbook

**Do You Want To Lose Weight & Transform Your Body?**

## It's Never Too Late To Start Intermittent Fasting & Shed Those Stubborn Extra Pounds!

If you are looking for a simple and effective weight loss strategy that will allow you to lose weight without counting calories or starving, then this the cookbook you NEED.

Unlike all those other fad diets that promise you the world and never deliver, intermittent fasting is here to change the way you approach your diet and perceive your lifestyle.

## Are You Ready To Reboot Your Diet?

In this foolproof weight loss cookbook, you will discover mouth-watering, healthy, easy, and budget-friendly recipes, including:

- Healthy, Quick & Delicious Breakfast
- Mouth-watering Lunch Recipes
- Effortless Dinner Meals
- Yummy Spaghetti, Soups, Sauces, Pizzas & More
- Top Recipes to Die for...

and much more!

Start Enjoying The Immense Health Benefits Of Intermittent Fasting While Enjoying Amazing Tastes.

ISBN 978-1-80307-441-2

90000

9 781803 074412

**DIET ACCLAIMED PRESS**

# Amazing Stories

# From

# New Brunswick

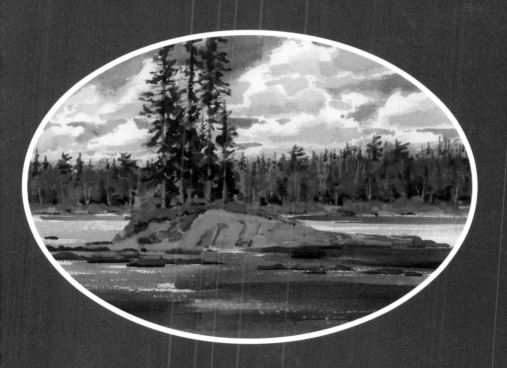

# PETER D. CLARK